IMPACTS OF GREEN MEDITERRANEAN DIET ON WEIGHT LOSS

Exploring the richness of Mediterranean diets

By

Dr DOUGLAS JASON

TABLE OF CONTENT

ABOUT THE AUTHOR

INTRODUCTION

TABLE OF CONTENT

IMPACTS OF GREEN MEDITERRANEAN DIET ON WEIGHT LOSS

Exploring the richness of Mediterranean diets

INTRODUCTION

Chapter 1
contrasts the green and traditional MED diets.

CHAPTER 2.
THE GREEN MED DIET IS ENRICHED WITH ENOUGH POLYPHENOLS.

CHAPTER 3.
The green MED diet's health advantages.

CHAPTER 4.
THE POLYPHENOL LEVEL IN GREEN MEDIEVAL DIET IS HIGHER.

CONCLUSION

ABOUT THE AUTHOR

Dr. Douglas Jason is a certified dietician who has a strong passion for wellness and a big eagerness to help people all over the world. He uses healthy food, herbs, spices, and other useful tools to help mankind realize its overall goal of optimum health.

INTRODUCTION

According to a recent study, the green version of the popular eating plan decreases visceral fat by 14%, which is twice as much as the standard form.

According to a recent study, the "green" Mediterranean diet significantly reduced visceral fat by 14%, which is twice as much as the traditional Mediterranean diet's (MED) 7% reduction.

A lower chance of developing diabetes, cardiovascular disease, depression, and cognitive decline are some advantages of the green MED diet.

Additionally demonstrated to lower blood pressure and cholesterol, the green MED diet may offer greater protection against age-related brain atrophy than the standard MED diet. Experts assert that polyphenols are crucial to the success of the green MED diet.
Visceral fat is abdominal fat that collects in the middle of the stomach. The kidneys, pancreas, and liver are all encased in this kind of fat.

Your health can be harmed by excess visceral fat, which can also cause diabetes, dementia, and heart disease.

Adopting healthier eating habits is one of the best methods to minimize visceral fat. Nutritionists frequently suggest the Mediterranean diet (MED), which has been named the greatest diet in the world for five years running.

The idea of a "green" Mediterranean diet was suggested in 2020 by the DIRECT PLUS research group.

Compared to the conventional MED diet, green MED comprises more plant-based meals and less meat. The DIRECT PLUS researchers found that the MED diet had many health advantages, from enhancing gut health to lowering the chance of developing age-related degenerative diseases.

Now, a new study indicated that, when compared to the standard Mediterranean diet (7%) and a healthy diet (4.5%), the green Mediterranean diet reduced visceral fat by the most 14%.

The outcomes provide more proof that the green MED diet may be even healthier than the conventional one.

Chapter 1

contrasts the green and traditional MED diets.

The green Mediterranean diet fully forbids red and processed meats, whereas the traditional Mediterranean diet occasionally permits certain foods. This is one of the main differences between the two diets.

The green MED diet places a greater emphasis on plant-based proteins than the standard MED diet, according to Mackenzie Burgess, RDN, a registered dietitian nutritionist and recipe developer at

Cheerful Choices in Fort Collins, Colorado.

Another distinction is that the green MED diet calls for the daily consumption of green tea, walnuts, and Mankai duckweed (an aquatic plant abundant in protein), all of which have high levels of beneficial polyphenols.

Burgess said that the green MED diet has more structure than the Mediterranean diet because it specifies the number of calories, grams of protein, and specific items to eat each day.

The current research indicates that the green form of the MED diet may be even more effective for preventing or controlling chronic diseases, even though both variants of the MED diet contain anti-inflammatory and antioxidant items.

The aquatic duckweed plant, used as a meat replacement in the study, may be one contributing reason. The duckweed plant is rich in bioavailable protein, iron, B12, vitamins, minerals, polyphenols, and other nutrients that are all known to have health advantages.

CHAPTER 2.

THE GREEN MED DIET IS ENRICHED WITH ENOUGH POLYPHENOLS.

According to study author Hila Zelicha RD, Ph.D., clinical dietitian and postdoctoral fellow at the Department of General Surgery at the University of California Los Angeles, "the green Mediterranean diet group was enriched with polyphenols compounds in various plant-based foods and have potential antioxidant and antiinflammatory roles in the prevention and management of several diseases, such as cardiovascular, hypertension, diabetes, and Alzheimer's disease."

CHAPTER 3.

The green MED diet's health advantages.

Similar health advantages to those of the standard MED diet are provided by the green MED diet, including:

lower likelihood of developing chronic illness
better blood pressure levels reduced cholesterol
According to a 2021 study, the green MED diet may offer some extra advantages over the traditional MED diet, such as:

reduced waist measurement
lower levels of LDL (bad) cholesterol
decreasing the diastolic blood
pressure
Burgess noted that the advantages
might also include lessened DNA
damage and a decreased risk of
melancholy and cognitive decline,
despite the fact that research on the
green MED diet is still in its infancy.

According to a 2022 study, the
green MED diet's high polyphenol
content made it more protective
against age-related brain shrinkage.

Polyphenols' effects on weight loss
Many foods made from plants
include polyphenols.

The green MED diet's effects on polyphenols can lead to a faster fatty acid breakdown and increased energy expenditure, which may ultimately have an impact on the amount of fat formation.

Yes, polyphenols did aid with visceral fat reduction.

Nutritionists concur that polyphenols may aid in the prevention and treatment of obesity as well as weight loss.

CHAPTER 4.

THE POLYPHENOL LEVEL IN GREEN MEDIEVAL DIET IS HIGHER.

According to Burgess, the new study demonstrates that participants in the green Mediterranean diet group had higher levels of polyphenols in their plasma and urine as a result of consuming green tea, walnuts, and duckweed powder, which may help to explain why this group experienced a greater reduction in visceral fat.

The link between polyphenols and lower visceral fat is supported by additional research on the polyphenols present in tea and olives.

Through a number of processes, the high level of polyphenols in a green MED diet is probably causing lower visceral fat.

polyphenols may reduce chronic inflammation, boost glucose uptake into muscles, prevent the formation of new blood vessels in adipose tissue, and restrict the absorption of fat after eating.

Additionally, food is the greatest way to consume polyphenols as opposed to supplements. Polyphenol-rich foods include:

grapes and berries
Red onion, spinach, coffee, tea,
cocoa, herbs, and spices
olives\snuts

CONCLUSION

According to recent studies, the classic Mediterranean diet reduced visceral fat by 7%, the healthy diet by 4.5%, and the green Mediterranean diet by the greatest (14%).

The green MED diet has numerous health advantages, some of which may outweigh those of the standard MED diet.

Reduced risk of diabetes, cardiovascular disease, depression, and cognitive decline are some of these advantages. The green MED diet has the potential to be more effective than the standard MED diet at lowering blood pressure and cholesterol levels, as well as protecting against age-related brain atrophy.

According to the current study, polyphenols are an important component of the green MED diet that has positive health impacts, especially when it comes to fat loss.

Ask your healthcare provider or a trained dietitian for more information if you're curious about how the green MED diet can improve your health.